Killer Diabetes – Heal by Yourself

Vivek Kamath

ISBN:1522872393
ISBN-13:9781522870395

ACKNOWLEDGEMENT

I am grateful to my mother Late Mrs. Vimala Kamath for giving me the birth because of which I am able to attain this great moment of writing a book on Killer Diabetes Heal by Yourself. My Mother died of Diabetes and Cardiac Aliment way back in November 2006. Today I am able to cure Diabetes, Heart Aliment thru Reiki healing method and many other diseases without Medicines. It was unfortunate that I do not have my mother with me. I am sure her departed soul will now be able to rest in peace today by seeing the achievement of her beloved son. My mother's love and affection was a key for me to attain this position today and instrumental in shaping up my life and destiny. I am very thankful to my mother for giving me this great opportunity to serve the world.

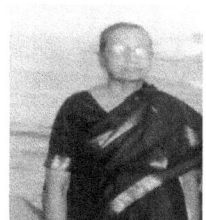

I would like to express my gratitude and heart-full of love to great Reiki Guru and Founder Dr Mikao Usui of Japan.

I would like to thank myself because of my inner strength with which I could able to convert the difficult situations or challenges faced in my life as a great opportunity for learning and always believed that life is a continuous education process. Furthermore, I strongly believed in my life that whatever happens in life it will happen for a good cause and these are based on our good and bad karma/action of past and current life.

CONTENTS

1 Introduction

Background about the Author

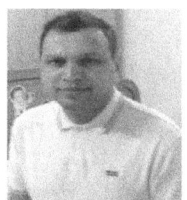

Author Vivek Kamath is an Indian Software Engineer by profession. Author has worked with the world's top International Banks across the globe for nearly 20 years to manage large scale Information Technology (IT) projects. Author is also a Reiki Healing Master Cum Practitioner and Practicing Reiki Healing, Mexican Healing, Crystal Healing, Melchizedek Method of healing from the last 5 years. Author has healed many diabetic patients, blood pressure patients (both high and low blood pressure), Heart Patients (removed the heart blocks), removed kidney stones , cured sinusitis, severe joint pains, constipation, migraines, headaches, insomnia, stomach related problems, diabetic gum problems, skin problems (dry skin, eczema) and chronic nasal allergies, nasal blockages without any medicines. Some of the above treatments have been completed within a week to maximum 1 month duration. Author has intention to help as much as diabetic patients to come out of the disease without any medicines. Author has an intention to build a healing center for diabetic patients across the globe.

For whom was this book prepared?

This book intended for people who are Type1, Type2 Diabetic Patients and Pre Diabetic Patients. The calorie management for European, British, American, Mexican, Italian, Asian Food, North and South Indian Food diet included in the Appendixes. Author intends to release to separate book for China Diabetic Patients in Mandarin Language covering the Chinese Herbs and other in-country specific treatments as China has the world's highest number of diabetic patients (98.4 million).

This book covers diabetic history, key finding across the globe, causes, symptoms, medicines, herbal remedies, and various healing techniques to cure diabetes without any medicines. This book is intended to help diabetic patients to follow the daily meal menu timetable various exercises, Yoga, travel checklist, precautions to be taken against the Killer Disease Diabetes.

It is primarily aimed to control the blood glucose level with the proper food diet, weight management and practicing any of the healing methods provided in the book. The objective is to assist the diabetic patients to come out of Life term dependency on Allopathic medicines and allopathic medicines side effects which are quite dangerous for long term life. The side effects of one of the diabetes drug (metformin) and the impact of metformin taking with other allopathic drugs have been highlighted in this book. (Section 7J)

This book should help the diabetic patients to come out of diabetic disease within 3 months of practicing any one of the healing method given in the section 7 of this book plus following the weight management techniques (food and exercise/workout) and practicing effective stress management techniques.

Author has personally healed himself and several of his patients who were having high fasting glucose and insulin dependent patients using Reiki and Crystal healing method. Some of the patients have been completely cured and they were able to maintain a normal blood glucose level within a month. All these patients were consuming allopathic medicines for more than 2 decades. Author has used distant healing method (Patients can reside far away from the healer) of Reiki to heal some of the patients. Distant healing has been found to be very effective.

What is Diabetes and Types of Diabetes?

Diabetes (diabetes mellitus) is classed as a metabolism disorder. Metabolism meaning our way our bodies use digested food for energy and growth. Most of what we eat is broken down into glucose.

What Is Glucose?

Glucose is the simple sugar that is the chief source of energy. Glucose is found in the blood and is the main sugar that the body manufactures. The body makes glucose from all three elements of food protein, fats, and carbohydrates but the largest amount of glucose derives from carbohydrates. Glucose serves as the major source of energy for living cells. However, cells cannot use glucose without the help of insulin. Also known as dextrose

What Is Insulin?

Insulin is a hormone that is produced by the pancreas. After eating, the pancreas automatically releases an adequate quantity of insulin to move the glucose present in our blood into the cells, as soon as glucose enters the cells blood-glucose levels drop.

How and Where Insulin is produced in the Body?

Insulin is a hormone made up of a small polypeptide protein that is secreted by the pancreas, which acts as both an endocrine and exocrine gland. Endocrine glands are the system of glands that secrete hormones to regulate body functions. Exocrine glands aid in digestion.

The pancreas sits behind the stomach, nestled in the curve of the duodenum (the first part of the small intestine), and clusters of cells called islets of Langerhans. Islets are made up of beta cells, which produce and release insulin into the bloodstream. A below picture shows the location of Pancreas in our human body.

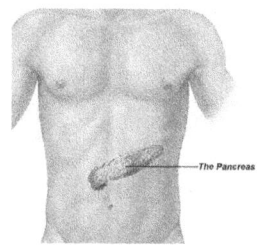

Types of Diabetes

Type 1 Diabetes

Type 1 diabetes is a disorder in which the pancreas can no longer produce insulin. It is called as juvenile diabetes. It is sometimes referred to as insulin-dependent diabetes mellitus.

Type1 Pancreas Function

1. Stomach converts food into glucose
2. Glucose enters the blood vessel
3. Pancreas produce no insulin
4. Glucose builds up in the blood stream

Type 2 Diabetes

In type 2 diabetes, the pancreas can produce insulin, but it may not be enough. Some people produce insulin, but the body doesn't use it effectively. Some, but not all people with type 2 diabetes need to take insulin. Most of the time, the disease can be successfully managed with treatment and healthy lifestyle choices. Below diagram shows the difference between normal pancreas function vs Type1 Diabetes and Type2 Diabetes.

Type 2 Pancreas Function

1. Stomach and Small Intestine break down food into glucose

2. Glucose enter the blood stream

3. Gastric Hormones promote Insulin secretion in response to Glucose

4. Pancreas produces insulin. Body is resistant to its effect

5. Glucose builds up in the blood vessel damaging blood vessel.

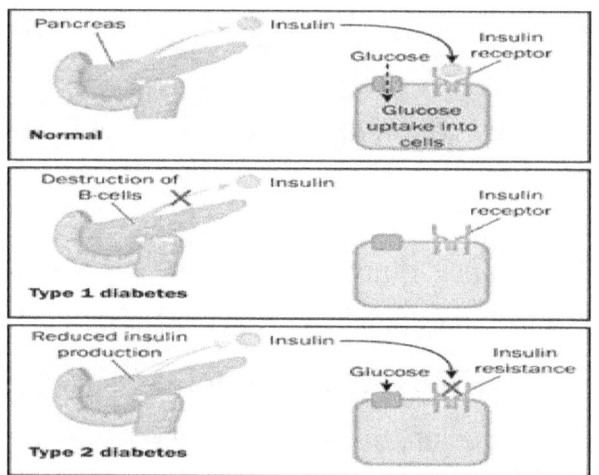

Gestational Diabetes

Gestational diabetes is diabetes that develops during pregnancy. According to the National Institute of Diabetes Digestive Kidney Diseases (NIDDK , women with gestational diabetes have a 35 to 60 percent chance of developing type 2 diabetes within 20 years.

Prediabetes

Blood glucose levels are higher than they should be, but not high enough to qualify as diabetes, you have prediabetes. Prediabetes puts you at increased risk of type 2 diabetes. In many cases, changes in diet and exercise can delay or prevent onset of the disease.

2 History of Diabetes

Diabetes was one of the first diseases described, with an Egyptian manuscript from 1500.

For 2,000 years, diabetes has been recognized as a devastating, deadly and Killer disease. Diabetes comes from Greek, and it means a "siphon". Aretus the Cappadocian, a Greek physician during the second century A.D., named the condition *diabainein*. He described patients who were passing too much water (polyuria) - like a siphon. The word became "diabetes" from the English adoption of the Medieval Latin diabetes.

In 1675, Thomas Willis added mellitus to the term, although it is commonly referred o as diabetes. *Mel* in

Latin means "honey"; the urine and blood of people with diabetes has excess glucose, and glucose is sweet like honey. Diabetes mellitus could literally mean "siphoning off sweet water".

Type 1 and Type 2 diabetes were identified as separate conditions for the first time by the Indian physicians Sushruta and Charaka in 400-500 CE with type 1 associated with youth and type 2 with being overweight

Year of Development	Description of the Research
1921/ 1922	Canadians Frederick Banting and Charles Herbert Best isolated and purified insulin
1935	Roger Hinsworth discovered there were two types of diabetes "insulin sensitive type1 and "insulin sensitive type 2"
1938	NPH insulin was first marketed across the globe

1950	Oral medications called sulfonylureas were developed for people with type 2 diabetes. These drugs stimulate the pancreas to produce more insulin, helping people with type 2 keep tighter control over their blood sugars.
1970	The insulin pump was designed to mimic the body's normal release of insulin.
1979	The hemoglobin A1c test was devised in order to create a more precise blood sugar measurement. The A1c became a standard measurement for blood sugar control in the comprehensive ten-year study from 1983 to 1993: the Diabetes Control and Complications Trial (DCCT).
1995	Metformin, an oral medication for people with type 2 diabetes, was finally approved for use inthe United States by the FDA. Unlike sulfonylurea drugs, which stimulate insulin release, metformin does not increase insulin production. Instead, it heightens sensitivity to insulin and increases the muscles' ability to use the insulin. Because metformin promotes weight loss, decreases

hyperglycemia, and improves lipid levels, it is an effective tool for people with type 2 diabetes when used in conjunction with sulfonylureas.

1995   Precose, an oral medication, was approved for use by people with type 2 diabetes. Precose delays the digestion of carbohydrates, thereby reducing the sudden rise in blood glucose after eating a meal.

1996   Lispro, a new fast-acting insulin, was released by Eli Lilly under the brand name Humalog. Lispro is designed to simulate the body's natural insulin output. Because of lispro's fast-acting tendencies, patients can take this insulin 15 minutes or less before eating a meal, instead of waiting as they would with Regular insulin.

3 Diabetic Key Findings across the world

1. Type 2 diabetes is on the rise worldwide. The International Diabetes Federation (IDF) reports that as of 2013 there were more than 387 million people living with diabetes

2. The World Health Organization (WHO) estimates that 90 percent of people around the world who suffer from diabetes suffer from type 2 diabetes.

3. In 2004, high blood sugar as a result of diabetes led to an estimated 3.4 million deaths worldwide

4. More than eight of every 10 diabetes-related deaths occur in low- and middle-income countries

5. In developing nations, more than half of all diabetes cases go undiagnosed

6. World Health Organization (WHO) anticipates that worldwide deaths attributable to diabetes will double by 2030

7. Adults ages 40 to 59 comprise the world's age group with the highest diabetes rates, although this is expected to shift to adult ages 60 to 79 by 2030

8. In 2014 the global prevalence of diabetes was estimated to be 9% among adults aged 18+ years

9. In 2012, an estimated 1.5 million deaths were directly caused by diabetes

10. More than 80% of diabetes deaths occur in low- and middle-income countries

11. WHO projects that diabetes will be the 7th leading cause of death in 2030

12. Healthy diet, regular physical activity, maintaining a normal body weight and avoiding tobacco use can prevent or delay the onset of type 2 diabetes

Snapshot of Diabetes across the World Country Wise

Country	Patients in Million
China	98.4
India	65.5
USA	24.4
Brazil	11.9
Russia	10.9
Mexico	8.7
Indonesia	8.5
Germany	7.6
Egypt	7.5
Japan	7.2

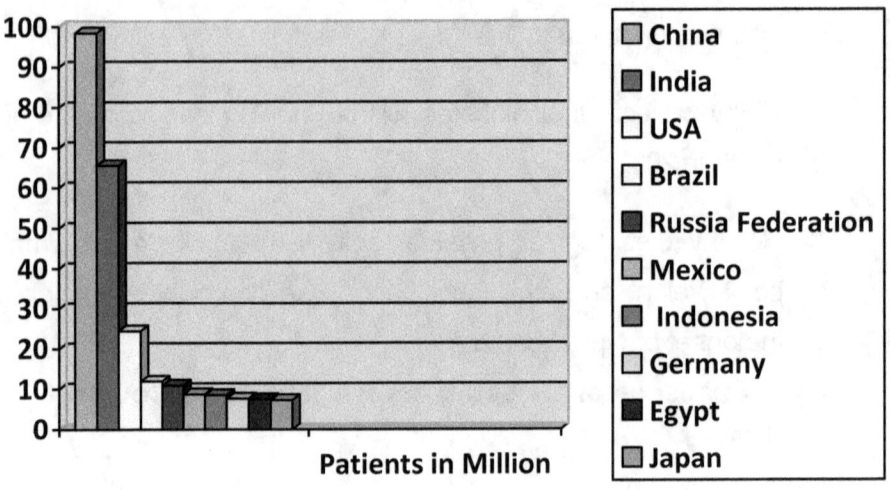

Patients in Million

- China
- India
- USA
- Brazil
- Russia Federation
- Mexico
- Indonesia
- Germany
- Egypt
- Japan

Snapshot of Diabetes across the World by Region Wise

Region	Diabetic Patients in Million
North America and Caribbean	39
Europe	52
Middle East and North Africa	37
South East Asia	75
Western Pacific	138
South and Central America	25
Africa	22

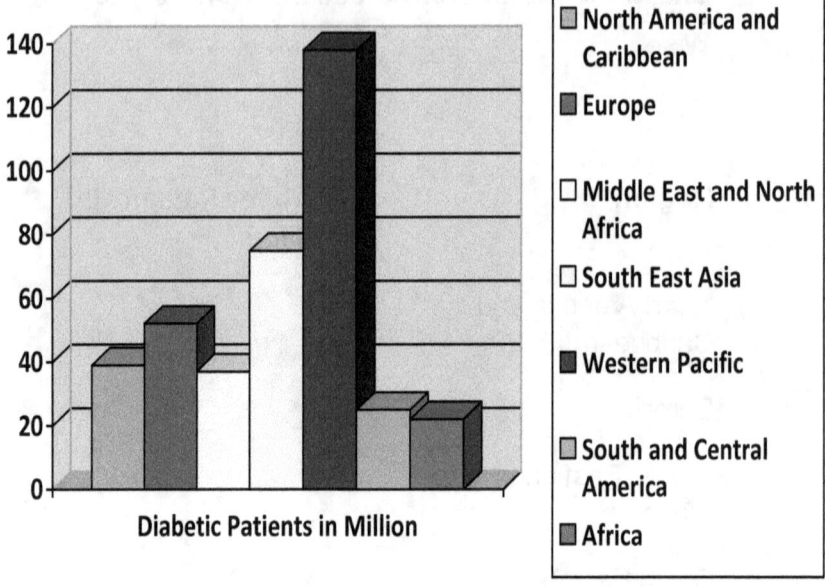

Diabetic Patients in Million

Legend:
- North America and Caribbean
- Europe
- Middle East and North Africa
- South East Asia
- Western Pacific
- South and Central America
- Africa

4 Complication of Diabetes

Following are the common complications of uncontrolled diabetes.

1. **Heart problems** - such as ischemic heart disease, when the blood supply to the heart muscle is diminished

2. **Hypertension** - common in people with diabetes, which can raise the risk of kidney disease, eye problems, heart attack and stroke

3. **Mental health** - uncontrolled diabetes raises the risk of suffering from depression, anxiety and some other mental disorders

4. **Eye complications** – glaucoma, cataracts, diabetic retinopathy, and some others.

5. **Foot complications** - neuropathy, ulcers, and sometimes gangrene which may require that the foot be amputated

6. **Skin complications** - people with diabetes are more susceptible to skin infections and skin disorders

7. **Hearing loss** - diabetes patients have a higher risk of developing hearing problems

8. **Gum disease** - there is a much higher prevalence of gum disease among diabetes patients

9. **Gastroparesis** - the muscles of the stomach stop working properly

10. **Ketoacidosis** - a combination of ketosis and acidosis; accumulation of ketone bodies and acidity in the blood.

11. **Neuropathy** - diabetic neuropathy is a type of nerve damage which can lead to several different problems.

12. **HHNS (Hyperosmolar Hyperglycemic Nonketotic Syndrome)** - blood glucose levels shoot up too high, and there are no ketones present in the blood or urine. It is an emergency condition.

13. **Nephropathy** - uncontrolled blood pressure can lead to kidney disease

14. **PAD (peripheral arterial disease)** - symptoms may include pain in the leg, tingling and sometimes problems walking properly

15. **Stroke** - if blood pressure, cholesterol levels, and blood glucose levels are not controlled, the risk of stroke increases significantly

16. **Erectile dysfunction** - male impotence.

17. **Infections** - people with badly controlled diabetes are much more susceptible to infections

18. **Healing of wounds** - cuts and lesions take much longer to heal

5 Symptoms of Diabetes

Individuals can experience different signs and symptoms of diabetes, and sometimes there may be no signs. Some of the signs commonly experienced has been shown in the below table.

1   Increase in Hunger

2   Excessive Thirst

3   Frequent Urination

4   Fatigue and Tiredness

5   Lack of Concentration

6   Weight Loss

7   Frequent Infections

8   Reduced Immunity which may include delay

          in healing wounds or any other disease

          Sexual Dysfunction

10   Stomach Pain and Vomiting

11   Numbness in Feet

The development of type 1 diabetes is usually sudden and dramatic while the symptoms can often be mild or absent in people with type 2 diabetes, making this type of diabetes hard to detect. There may not be any symptoms for pre-diabetes patients.

6 Causes of Diabetes

It is still not clear the real causes of killer diabetes diseases. There are considerable researches going on across the globe to check the real causes of diabetes.

Research and Cost Spending on Diabetes

In 2015, Diabetes Australia has committed more than $3.8 million to diabetes research projects. Over the past eight years, the Diabetes Australia Research Program has invested $23 million in 335 diabetes research projects across Australia

The American Diabetes Association (Association) released new research on March 6, 2013 estimating the total costs of diagnosed diabetes have risen to $245 billion in 2012.

A report published in the journal Diabetic Medicine UK has projected that the NHS's (National Health Services) annual spending on diabetes in the UK will increase from £9.8 billion to £16.9 billion over the next 25 years..

Potential Causes of Diabetes

Combination of genetic susceptibility and environmental factors, though exactly what many of those factors are is still unclear. It is known that our immune system which normally fights harmful bacteria or viruses attacks and destroys our insulin production cells in the pancreas. This leaves us with little or no insulin instead of being transported into our cells, sugar builds up in our bloodstream. This is the case normally in Type1 diabetes. However, in Type 2 Diabetes, being overweight is strongly linked to development of type2 diabetes but not everyone with type 2 diabetes is overweight.

7 Tests for Diabetes

1. **Fasting Plasma Glucose (FPG) test:** It is used to measure blood sugar level after the person has been fasting for at least 8 hours.

2. **Oral glucose tolerance test (OGTT):** Like the fasting plasma glucose test, this test also requires 8 hours of fasting. Following that, you have to drink a glass of water mixed with 75g of glucose. The blood glucose is then checked after 2 hours of taking the glucose water.

3. **HbA1C test or glycated hemoglobin test:** This test is specifically used to diagnose type 2 diabetes. It is also used to check overall regulation of blood sugar and to check if the treatment given for reducing blood sugar is effective. It measures the amount of sugar or glucose attached to hemoglobin in red blood cells (RBCs) circulating the body. Because the average life of a RBC is 100-120 days, blood sugar detected with this test reflects a person's sugar level over the period of three months.

Test Results Range

Normal

Fasting Plasma Glucose (Mg/Dl) Below 100

Oral Glucose Tolerance Test (mg/Dl) Below 140

HbA1C (%) Below 5.7

Prediabetes

Fasting Plasma Glucose (Mg/Dl) Between 100 and 125

Oral Glucose Tolerance Test (mg/Dl) Between 140 and 199

HbA1C (%) Between 5.7 and 6.4

Diabetes

Fasting Plasma Glucose (Mg/Dl) Above 125

Oral Glucose Tolerance Test (mg/Dl) 200 and Above

HbA1C (%) Above 5.7

8 Cure for diabetes

Following are some of the Healing for Diabetes.

A.   Reiki Healing

Reiki is a form of alternative medicine developed in 1922 by Japanese Buddhist Dr. Mikao Usui.

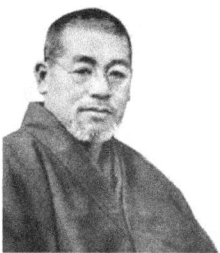

Mikao Usui 臼井甕男(1865–1926)

It uses a technique commonly called palm healing or hands-on-healing.The word Reiki is made of two Japanese words – Rei which means "God's Wisdom or the Higher Power" and Ki which means "life force energy". So Reiki is actually "spiritually guided life force energy or universal energy".

Diabetes can be completely healed using Reiki Healing. Distant Healing (Patients need not be present in the physical location of the healer/Reiki Practitioner) method found to be very effective.

B.   Pranic Healing®

Pranic Healing® is a simple yet powerful & effective system of no-touch energy healing. It is based on the fundamental principles that the body is a *self-repairing* living entity that possesses the ability to heal itself and that the healing process is accelerated by increasing this life force that is readily available from the sun, air and ground to address physical & emotional imbalances. Pranic Healing® requires no drugs, gadgets, not even physical contact with the subject. Physical contact is not required because the practitioner is working on the bioplasmic or energy body/aura of the person and not directly on the physical body. It is the energy body that absorbs life energy and distributes it throughout the physical body, to the muscles, organs, glands, etc. The reason Pranic Healing® works on the energy body is that physical ailments first appear as energetic disruptions in the aura before manifesting as problems in the physical body. Diabetes can be cured completely by Pranic Healing.

C.   Mexican Healing

Mexican Healing is a Powerful Egyptian healing technique to remove black magic, critical   ailments, curse, cleanse past life Karmas. Light energy is used to here to heal the patients.

This healing technique can be used to heal diabetes. Diabetes can be completely healed by healing Pancreas and Solar plexus Chakra using Mexican Healing Technique.

D.   Crystal Healing

A method of healing with the use of crystals placed on or around the body is called Crystal Healing. Crystal help in releasing and clearing negative energy from the human body. Each crystal has a unique internal structure, which causes it to resonate at a certain frequency. It is this resonance that is said to give crystals their healing abilities.

The human body has a complex electromagnetic system, also known as a vibrational energy system. Nature has created crystals to be perfect electromagnetic conductors, capable of interacting with our electromagnetic system. Crystals have been found to carry vibration that activates certain energy centers within our electromagnetic system, thus having a positive effect on our entire body systems. Chakras are the spinning wheels of conscious energy. There are 7 major chakras and 50 minor chakras. Chakras absorb the universal energy or Prana. In Crystal Healing, crystals must be placed on the chakra of the human body. The colours of the crystals are associated with the various chakra centers in the body. Each chakra has a color and if crystals of the same colour are placed on the associated center, it affects that area of the body. When crystals are placed at corresponding chakra point, they cleanse and energize the chakra. For Diabetes Healing, 3rd Chakra – Solar Plexus needs to be healed. Citrine, Amber and Topaz are the crystals can be used to heal the Solar Plexus Chakra.

E.   The Melchizedek Method – Holographic Healing

The Melchizedek Method is systematic approach to eternal health. It is using Holographic Healing technique. The whole universe was born through the scattered sphere called "The Hologram of Love It is the sacred sphere of unconditional love and sacred geometric pattern which gave birth to whole universe. Our   DNA, RNA, was born through this holographic pattern. The finest particle of our atomic cell structure has pattern within it. Healing is amazingly simple, quick and very effective. All Diseases, body and mental malfunction can be approached and healed permanently with no limitation to implementation. The Melchizedek Method demonstrates and teaches the skill of removing any part of the body, outer bodies and thought programming into the higher dimensions to be cleansed and healed and then returned into the physical completely perfect. Holographic healing and rejuvenation is a skill all human beings will practice in the future, and will be instrumental in ridding the planet of illness and disease. To cure Diabetes using Melchizedek Method, the entire endocrine system hologram needs to be plugged out from holographic body computer. The whole endocrine system hologram can be cleansed. Below is the Picture of Hologram of Love.

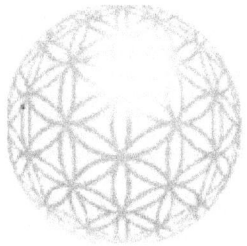

F.   Yoga

Yoga is Physical, mental and spiritual practice or discipline which originated in India. Yoga Gurus from India introduced yoga to the western countries.

In 1980's yoga became popular as a system of physical exercise across the western world. Yoga in Indian Traditions, however is more than physical exercise, it has a meditative and spiritual core. Following are the four Types of the Yoga need to be carried out to control diabetes. A detailed step to perform below 4 yoga has been provided in Appendix B.

Vrikshasana

It helps to stimulate the hormonal secretion of the pancreas

Dhanurasana

This yoga improves the functioning of pancreas and intestines. Thus helps in controlling blood sugar levels.

Organs like liver, pancreas and enzyme producing organs will function actively by practicing this asana.

Halasana

It stimulates the pancreas, spleen and activates immune system by massaging all the internal organs including pancreas. It improves kidney and liver functioning and strengthens the abdominal muscles. It also rejuvenates the mind.

Ardha Matsyendrasana

This asana massages the kidneys, pancreas, small intestines, gall bladder and liver, helping to stimulate digestion and squeeze out toxins. This yoga is very useful for diabetics, with concentration on the pancreas. It Increases the elasticity of the spine, tones the spinal nerves

G.   Mudra

The 5 yoga mudras for diabetes that every diabetic should know are:

Surya Mudra [Sun Mudra]: 'Surya' is a Sanskrit word that means 'Sun'. This mudra is known to increase the fire within the human body that in turn ensures a better metabolic rate. Diabetics, in general, have poor metabolic rates which results in increased sugar levels and weight gain.

Regular practice of this mudra will help boost

metabolic rates, thus ensuring loss of weight and lowering of sugar levels. The mudra also helps easing indigestion and associated problems

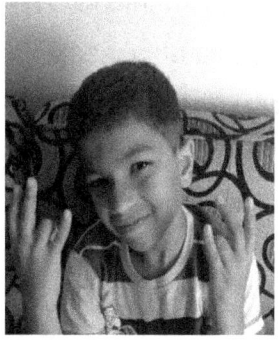

Pran Mudra

Improving the vital force of life and activates your Mooladhara Chakra or root chakra. Thus, it empowers you wholly within. The mudra, when practiced without fail, helps in detoxifying your body. Practicing this mudra alongside Apan Mudra has been proven to offer relief to those suffering from diabetes.

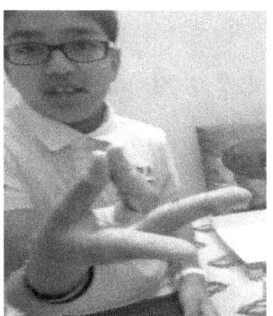

Apan Mudra [Mudra of Digestion]:

The mudra, also called the mudra of purification, is one of the easiest yoga mudras. It aids in striking a better balance between the elements within the human body. Thus, it ensures that the unwanted toxins are flushed out properly from your body. This mudra results in frequent urination for eliminating the wastes, thus lowering the blood sugar levels.

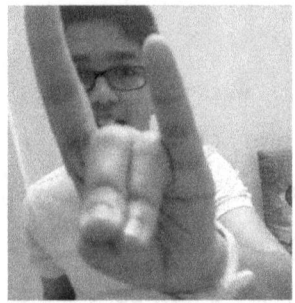

Gyan Mudra [Mudra of Knowledge]: Also known as Chin Mudra, it can be practiced by the diabetics to enjoy deep relaxation. It helps in relaxing the body and eliminating stress and other mind-related issues

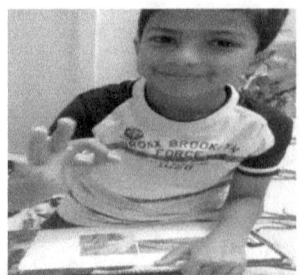

Linga Mudra Lingam, in Sanskrit, means phallus – the male reproductive organ. This mudra is helpful for those who are suffering from diabetes, but, indirectly. It helps in activating the fire element within the human body, thus generating intense heat. This, in turn, causes an increase in metabolic levels. The higher the metabolic levels, the more the chances of a person losing weight.

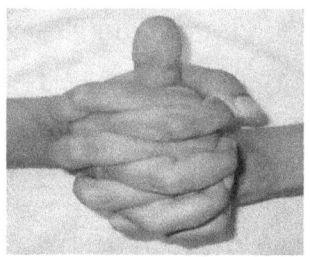

H.   Chanting of Mantras

What is Mantra?   Mantra means a sacred utterance, numinous sound, or a syllable world phonemes, or group of words believed by some to have psychological and spiritual power in Sanskrit Language   "Om Sri Lakshmi Narayana Namah" This mantra needs to be chanted 108 times on daily basis by keeping right hand on stomach immediately above navel and left hand on the right hand. This mantra activates the Solar Plexus Chakra of the Human body thereby activates the Pancreas to work effectively.

I. Homeopathic Medicines

Homeopathic medicines can helps in general health improvement in the diabetic persons.

If diabetes is treated in early stages with proper homeopathic treatment then the frequent fluctuations of blood sugar levels of diabetic individuals can be minimized effectively and even the use of anti-glycemic drugs or insulin can also be gradually reduced thereby ensuring long term benefit for the patient. Taking into consideration the psychological and the disease aspect of the patient according to principles of homeopathy, "GENETIC CONSTITUTIONAL THERAPY/TREATMENT" will be given to the patient to ensure maximum improvement in his/her general health without any side-effects

With the constitutional homeopathic treatment the decreased pancreatic secretion of insulin can be regained upto certain extent, thus ensuring blood glucose control in a natural manner.

With "constitutional homeopathic medicines" it is possible that patient does not get into complications of diabetes in their future like diabetic neuropathy, nephropathy or retinopathy etc.

J. Allopathic Medicines and side effects

Drug	Properties
Sulfonylureas	Increases the secretion of Insulin by the Pancreas
Biguanides	Inhibits glucose production by the liver and decreases insulin resistance
Thiazolidinediones	Decrease insulin resistance
Alpha-glucosidase Inhibitors	Delay absorption of glucose by the intestine
Meglitinides	Increases the secretion of Insulin by the Pancreas
Dipeptidyl peptidase 4 inhibitors	Promote the release of insulin from the pancreas after taking the meal.
Combination of sulfonylureas plus metformin	Increases the secretion of Insulin by the Pancreas. Inhibits glucose production by the liver and decreases insulin resistance

Side effects of Diabetic Allopathic Medicines – Metformin

I have only listed side effects of metformin drugs. There are side effects for all the diabetic allopathic drugs which I have not listed in this book. Also there are some side effects if the patients take metformin along with other allopathic medicines

Get emergency medical help if you have any of these signs of an allergic reaction to metformin: hives; difficult breathing; swelling of your face, lips, tongue, or throat.

This medication may cause lactic acidosis (a build-up of lactic acid in the body, which can be fatal). Lactic acidosis can start slowly and get worse over time. Get emergency medical help if you have even mild symptoms of lactic acidosis, such as:

1 Muscle pain or weakness

2 Numb or cold feeling in your arms and legs

3 Trouble Breathing

4 Feeling Dizzy, light-headed, tired or very weak

5 Stomach pain, nausea with vomiting or slow or uneven heart rate

6   Feeling short of breath even with mild exertion, swelling or rapid weight gain, fever, body aches and flu symptoms

Ayurveda Medicines

Ayurveda recognizes this disease right from the Vedic period with the name prameha. The word prameha denotes prabhuta mootrata (excessive urination) and aavila mootrata (turbid urine) and madhumeha means the flow of madhu (sugar) from the body. Depending on the physical constitution or body type (prakriti), or the health status of an individual, ayurvedic classics advocate two different types of therapy schedules for diabetics.

Apatarpana (de-nourishment) and Samshodhana (cleansing): This treatment is prescribed if you are obese and heavily   built. In this, along with anti-diabetic drugs, maximum stress is given on de-nourishment of fats and elimination of endotoxins by way of various exercises, fasting and cleansing manoeuvres known as panchakarma (five fold therapies viz. emesis, purgation, enema, blood letting and errhines).

Santarpana (replenishment) and Brumhana (body bulk promotion): This is   prescribed if you are chronically ill, with low immunity and underweight due to the draining of essential nutrients. This therapy helps in providing the easily acceptable nutrients and micronutrients to rebuild body tissues and help strengthen the defence mechanism without increasing circulating blood sugar, fats and other metabolites.

List of Herbs used for Diabetic Treatment in India. Ayurveda also recommends patients to perform Yoga, Mudras and try out the herbal home remedies for curing Diabetes. Jambhul (Eugenia jambolana) Powder from jamun core is useful.

1. Gurmar (gymnema sylvestre)

2. Bitter Gourd/bitter melon (Momordica charantia)

3. Bel (Aegle marmelos)

4. Fenugreek (Trigonella foenum graecum)

5. Turmeric

6. Neem

7. Triphala

8. Shilajit

Following are some of the Ayurveda Medicines used by Ayurveda Practitioners in India.

1. Chandrabrabha.

2. Arogyavardhini.

3. Asanad tablets

4. Shilajit Vati

5. Trivanga bhasma.

6. Vasant Kusumakar

Following table shows some of the very effective Home Remedies suggested by Ayurveda for s diabetic healing. These Remedies are slow compared to any other healing methods. But these home remedies have no side effects if you follow the usage of the doses. Anything excess is always bad for health.

Home Remedies

Description	Picture
Cinnamon has the ability to lower blood sugar levels by stimulating insulin activity. It has bioactive components which can reduce glucose level in the blood. Boil 2 or 3 sticks or 1 teaspoon powder in hot water and drink it on daily basis. Alternatively, we can use it with warm beverages, juices, smoothies or even in dishes. However, one should not use it	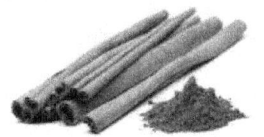

in excess as it can create lot of heat, burning in stomach sometimes in the body and it may increases the risk of liver damage.

- Mix one-half to one teaspoon of cinnamon in a cup of warm water. Drink it daily.

Bitter gourd can be helpful for controlling diabetes due to its blood glucose lowering effects. It helps increase pancreatic insulin secretion and prevents insulin resistance. Thus, bitter gourd is beneficial for both type 1 and type 2 diabetes. Drink some bitter gourd juice on an empty stomach each morning. Follow this treatment daily in the morning for at least few months.

-

Fenugreek is an herb that can also be used to control diabetes, improve glucose tolerance and lower blood sugar levels due to its hypoglycaemic activity. It also stimulates the secretion of glucose-dependent insulin. Being high in fiber, it slows down the absorption of carbohydrates and sugars. Soak two tablespoons of fenugreek seeds in water overnight. Drink the water along with the seeds in the morning on an empty stomach.

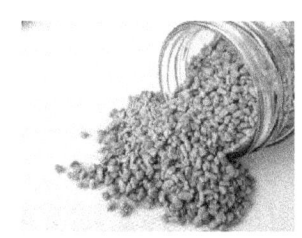

Indian gooseberry, also known as Amla, is rich in Vitamin C and Indian gooseberry juice promotes proper functioning of your pancreas. Grate 2 or 3 Indian gooseberries and mix with water and drink on daily basis.

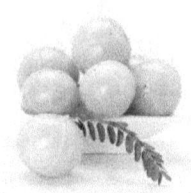

Okra, also called ladies' finger, has constituents such as polyphenolic molecules that can help reduce blood glucose levels and control diabetes.

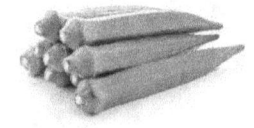

Knokol can be used as a salad in your daily meal or as a one of the snack. This vegetable high in fiber acts as an insulin to diabetic patients.

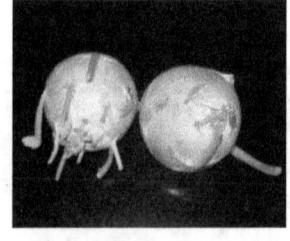

Black plum or

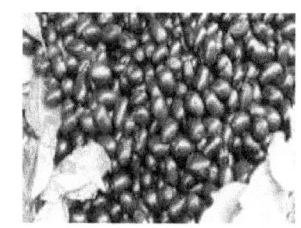

jambul, also known as jamun can help a lot in controlling blood sugar level because it contains anthocyanins, ellagic acid, hydrolysable tannins etc. In fact, research has shown that the fruits and seeds of this plant have hypoglycemic effects as they help reduce blood and urine sugar levels rapidly. The seeds, in particular, contain glycoside jamboline and alkaloid jambosine that regulate control blood sugar levels.

Mango Leaves
Soak 10 to 15 tender mango leave in a glass of water overnight. In the morning, filter the water

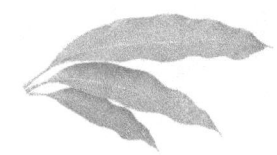

and drink it on an empty stomach. This can lower blood glucose level to some extent

Aloe vera gel helps lower fasting blood glucose levels. It contains phytosterols that have possible anti-hyperglycemic effects for type 2 diabetes.

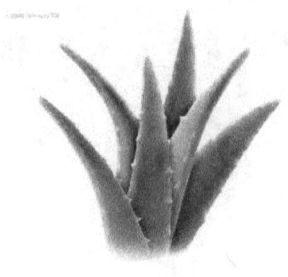

Guava due to its vitamin C and high fiber content eating guava can be really helpful in maintaining the blood glucose level.

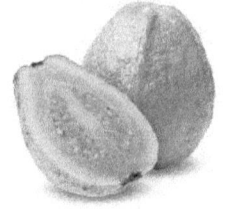

9 Food Time Table and List of Food To Be Avoided

Normally People take 3 large meals in a day and do not take any food in between the meals. The Gap between 3 large meals causes elevation of glucose in Diabetic Patients. Hence, it is advisable for diabetic patients to split these 3 large meals into 3 medium meals and 4 or 5 small snack meals to minimize the load on Pancreas and Liver. Please refer to total calorie needs to table in Appendix A based on your age, gender and activity level.

It is very important that one should have first meal/breakfast to be taken within 1 hour after waking up. Furthermore, Diabetic patients need to take a small snack before going to bed to keep the fasting blood glucose level normal. Make all the meals a low carbohydrate, low sugar, low fat, high fiber meal with little bit of protein Ideally the macronutrients carbohydrates, fat, and protein for adults above 18 years should get their calorie in the following percentage 45-65% from carbohydrates; 10-35% from protein; 20-25% from fats and fiber.

A Below Meal/Snack Time Table for Diabetic Patients.

Time	Meal/ Snack	Food/Juice	Calories
6:00 AM	Early Morning	Have a glass of Ladies Finger Juice (soaked overnight) along with 1 tea spoon of cinnamon powder.	20
7:00 AM	Breakfast – Meal 1	Make this as one of your big meal of the day. Balanced meal with Carbohydrate, Protein and low fat in the breakfast.	800
9:30 AM	Mid-Morning Snack 1	3 to 4 Small Slices of Papaya or low Glycemic load (GL) fruit. Please refer to list of fruits with Low Glycemic load.	80
11:30 AM	Snack 2	Small Portion of Vegetable Salad or Any Low fat Yoghurt	50
1:00 PM	Lunch – Meal 2	Balanced Meal. Non Vegetarian can add egg white or 1 slice of chicken or a fish in the meal. Avoid Deep fried food.	800
3:00 PM	Snack 3	2 Guava Fruit or 1 Apple or 1 cup of Yoghurt without added sugar	50

5:00 PM	Snack 4	1 cinnamon tea without sugar and 3 biscuits or 2 slice of wheat bread or 2 slice of wheat bread toast or 2 bread rusks.	50
7:30 PM	Dinner – Meal 3	Low Calorie Vegetarian Meal	500
9:30 PM	Light Snack 5	3 slices of apple or 2 almonds or 2 slices of papaya	50

The above table shows the Calorie requirement for a male aged between age 35 to 50 with moderate activities. Reducing 200 to 300 Calories in take can help to reduce the weight as a result of the weight loss, there could be significant reduction in glucose level can be observed. Also ensure Body Mass Index is in the healthy range. Please look into next page for some information on BMI and healthy range.

Food to Avoid for Diabetes

These top food offenders contain high amounts of fat, sodium, carbs, and calories that may increase your risk of high cholesterol, high blood pressure, heart disease, uncontrolled blood sugar, and weight gain.

Food	Food to be Avoided	Alternate Food
Anything highly processed, fried and made with white flour should be avoided	White Rice, White Bread and White Pasta/ Any fired items made of white flour	Brown Rice or Wild Rice or Wheat Pasta
Blended Coffees	These contains syrup, whipped cream and other topping can have lot of calories	Plain Coffee or Filter Coffee without Milk or Cream
Some Fruits contain more sugar	Bananas, Melons, Jackfruit, Mango, Peaches and nectarines	Papaya, Guava, Water Melon and fruits which are low in Glycemic index. Please refer to table or Appendix D fruits which are low

		glycemic value Glycemic Load. Glycemic Index is different from Glycemic Load.*
Fruit Juices, Fruit Smoothies	Avoid Fruit Juices available in the Super Market even if there are labels showing 'NO Added Sugar'.	Have fruits instead of having juices as it contains fiber. Eat fruits which has low glycemic load. Please refer to Appendix D for the list of fruits.
Refined Cereals	Sweetened breakfast cereals can cause elevation in glucose level in blood	Look for sugar free breakfast cereals or have protein meal for the breakfast.
Energy Bars	They may seem like a healthful snack choice, but many snack bars contain high levels of sugar and carbs, up to 450 calories and 60 grams of carbohydrates." Look for a balance of protein and carbs with a little fat (about 3 grams) and	Instead have low fat yoghurt or wheat sandwiches or wheat toast 2 slices.

	wholesome ingredients.	
Fatty Meat	Red Meat (Pork, Beef. Lamb)	Instead of this have white meat Chicken or Fish (Steamed Fish or Grilled or Baked Fish) Avoid Fried Fish or Chicken.
Pasta Sauce (Alfredo Sauce)	Alfredo Sauce is made from heavy cream, Parmesan Cheese and butter. This when we pour on white pasta total calorie of the meal can cross nearly 1000 calories. High fat, High Sodium sauce can elevate glucose easily.	Use Basil Sauce with less Cheese and low fat milk. Use Wheat Pasta.

Glycemic Index uses a scale from 0 to 100, where 100 is pure glucose. A food which has a high GI will cause a large increase in blood sugar, while a food with a lower GI will not have much impact at all. As a rough basis, mid-50s to mid-60s in a food's GI is considered average, while 70 and above is considered high. Foods with a GI of less than 55 are considered to have a low glycemic index, and thus will have smaller impact on blood sugar levels.

Glycemic load = GI/100 * Total grams of Carbohydrate

GL Range: A GL of above 20 is considered high, the 11-19 range is considered average, and below 11 is low.

What is BMI – Body Mass Index? BMI is a measure to see healthy weight based on individual's height and weight. Body Mass Index (BMI) is a person's weight in kilograms divided by the square of height in meters.

	BMI	Weight Classification
1	Less than 18.5	Under Weight
2	18.5 to 24.9	Healthy Weight
3	25 to 29.9	Overweight (Obese)

For better health and weight management, diabetic patients need to maintain BMI in the normal range (Healthy Weight Range BMI 18.5 to 24.9) by carrying out exercises recommended for diabetic patients and controlling the daily food calorie consumption regularly 80% glucose level can come down. The rest depends on stress management and their life style.

10 Workout or Exercise for Diabetes

People with diabetes are encouraged to exercise regularly for better blood sugar control and to reduce the risk of cardiovascular diseases. Muscle movement leads to greater sugar intake by muscle cells and lower blood sugar levels. Below is the list of workouts or exercises recommended for diabetes, however, it would be advisable to cross verify with your physician based on your age and other medical conditions.

1. Daily Brisk Walk from 30 to 45 minutes (Not Recommended for Patients with Heart Diseases)

2. Daily Moderate Walk of 30 to 45 minutes (those who have heart disease and Diabetes)

3. Yoga thrice a week (Check with your Physician people have heart or other aliment)

4. Light Jogging for 15 to 20 minutes weekly twice or thrice (Not Recommended for Patients have heart disease and diabetes)

5. Sports (Table Tennis, Tennis, Cricket, Base Ball, Badminton) 2 or 3 times a week

6. Rowing for 15 to 20 minutes thrice a week

7. Bicycling for 30 minutes thrice a week

Precautions one should take when it comes to exercise.

There are some exercise precautions which people with diabetes must take; however, when done safely, exercise is a valuable aid to optimal health.

Exercise precautions are designed to help people with diabetes avoid problems which can result from unwise exercise choices.

Hypoglycemia can occur if a person who is taking blood sugar lowering medication has:

1. Eaten too little carbohydrate (fruit, milk, starch) relative to the exercise.

2. Taken too much medication relative to the exercise

3. Combined effect of food and medication imbalances relative to the exercise

Those who do not take diabetes medication do not need to take these precautions. Drink plenty of water before, during and after exercise to stay well-hydrated.

Precautions for people on insulin or oral medication

Precautions to take if you take insulin or oral diabetes medication:

1. If your blood sugar level is less than 5.5 mmols/l (100 mg/dl) prior to exercise, take a carbohydrate snack prior to beginning the exercise.

2. If your blood sugar level is higher than 5.5 mmols/l (100 mg/dl) before exercise, it may not be necessary to take a carbohydrate snack before a light exercise session, but you may need extra carbohydrates during or following the exercise. Check your blood to see if your blood sugar dips below 4 mmols/l (70 mg/dl) following exercise.

3. If you experience hypoglycemia, follow the Carbohydrate Treatment guidelines. Follow up with your doctor. You may be advised to lower your medication on days you exercise if your blood sugar levels are well-controlled and usually within target range.

4. For long duration and/or high intensity exercise sessions, plan extra carbohydrate snacks during the activity. Additional carbohydrates are suggested each 30 to 60 minutes of exercise (e.g. soccer game, hiking, biking, skating, etc).

5. Always carry a fast-acting carbohydrate food such as glucose tablets when   exercising in the event blood sugar drops too low_and hypoglycemia symptoms develop during exercise.

6. Wear a form of ID, which identifies you as having diabetes, particularly if you are exercising alone so that others may help you appropriately in the event something unexpected happens.

11 Precautions for Diabetes Patients

1. Stress Management – Management of stress is a significant factor in Diabetes. The hormones your body may produce in response to prolonged stress may prevent insulin from working properly, which only makes matters worse

2. Stop or Reduce Alcohol Consumption: Alcohol can cause high or low blood sugar, depending on how much you drink and whether you eat at the same time. Manage your alcohol calorie in-take.

3. Stop or Reduce Smoking - Reduced blood flow in the legs and feet, which can lead to infections, ulcers and possible removal of a body part by surgery (amputation),heart disease, eye disease, stroke, Nerve damage and Kidney disease

4. Manage your blood pressure and Cholesterol – High blood pressure can damage blood vessels and high cholesterol can lead to heart attack and stroke

5. Keep an Eye on your Feet - High blood sugar can reduce blood flow and damage the nerves in your feet. Left untreated, cuts and blisters can lead to serious infections. Diabetes can lead to pain, tingling or loss of sensation in your feet. Take extra when you are changing your footwear. Avoid wearing shoes fitting very tight to your feet.

There are possibilities even after wearing socks you may get shoe boils.

6. Take Care of your Eyes - Your eye care specialist will check for signs of retinal damage, cataracts and glaucoma. Schedule 2 eye checkups for a year.

7. Visit your Dentist - Diabetes may leave you prone to gum infections. Brush your teeth at least twice a day, floss your teeth once a day and schedule dental exams at least twice a year. Visit your dentist if your gums bleed or look red or swollen.

8. Manage your Diet and Physical workout sessions

Please refer to Diabetic Food Chart Shown in section or check with Doctor for a suitable Diet plan and follow the physical exercise as per your suggestion from Physician based on your health fitness, medical conditions and age.

12 Check List for Diabetes Patients while Travelling

1. Take a reading of your glucose level in blood and urine before 2 or 3 days before your travel

2. Keep your Doctor's prescription, medical kit in one place. (In your hand bag if you are travelling by air) If you are taking a Insulin ensure you have cold pack with you. In case if you have uncontrolled or high diabetes you may need to inform the tour operator or neighbors sitting next to you in flight/bus/train.

3. Stick to your routine food time table provided in section 9 or the one which your doctor has provided to you.

4. Keep Glucose Tablets or Glucose Powder with you. You may need to prepare for low glucose strike due to increased physical activity during the sightseeing or walking etc.

5. Watch out the food you eat. If possible, check once in 2 days to test your blood glucose before and after the large meals to see how new foods are affecting your control.

6. If you are travelling by flight you may need doctor's letter to carry insulin and syringes before you onboard your

flight. Patients need to ensure what types and strengths of insulin are available in the place in which they will be travelling.

7. Insulin may be absorbed in warmer climates. Insulin should not be kept out of direct sunlight and kept cool.

13 Emergency Situation Management for Diabetes

The fluctuations in blood glucose levels can lead to a person with diabetic becoming unwell and losing consciousness. There are 2 conditions associated with diabetes.

1. Hyperglycaemia - high blood glucose

2. Hhypoglycaemia - low blood glucose

The more common emergency is hypoglycaemia which affects brain function and can lead to unconsciousness.

Hyperglycemia (high blood glucose) occurs when the body cannot produce any, or enough, insulin to regulate blood glucose. As a result,blood glucose levels become too high. This happens when there is no insulin to move glucose out of the bloodstream and into the cells to produce energy. The symptoms of hyperglycaemia are similar to the main symptoms of diabetes but they can come on suddenly and severely. If left untreated, hyperglycaemia can lead to diabetic ketoacidosis (DKA), which can eventually cause unconsciousness and even death. Hyperglycaemia can occur for several reasons including: a) eating too much b) steroid use e.g prednisolone and c) not taking diabetic medicines as prescribed by the doctor.

Hypoglycemia (low blood glucose)

People with type 2 diabetes who manage the condition with a combination of healthy eating and physical activity are not usually at risk of hypoglycaemia. If people are not taking any medications to lower their blood glucose levels, they don't tend to drop too low to cause a 'hypo' episode. Severe hypoglycemia is also very rare among people with type 2 diabetes who are taking blood glucose lowering medications such as metformin (Glucophage).

However people with type 2 diabetes who take medications that increase the amount of insulin released from the pancreas can be at risk of low blood glucose levels. These medications include Gliclazide, Glipizide and Glimpiride. Hypoglycemia also can happen in people with type 2 diabetes who use insulin.

14 Cure Diabetes without Medicines in Nut-Shell

Now, we have understood how we can cure diabetes. The below diagram explain the complete 360 degree cure in nut-shell. I have listed some basic principles of life for make it easy to heal yourself. .

Life is very simple do not make it very complicated. Just think that you came alone empty handed to this world and you are going to leave alone empty handed from this world.

Follow the basic principles of life documented in next page to overcome difficulty. I have taken some principles from few religions (Hindu, Christianity, Islam, Jain and Buddhism) Please refer to next page.

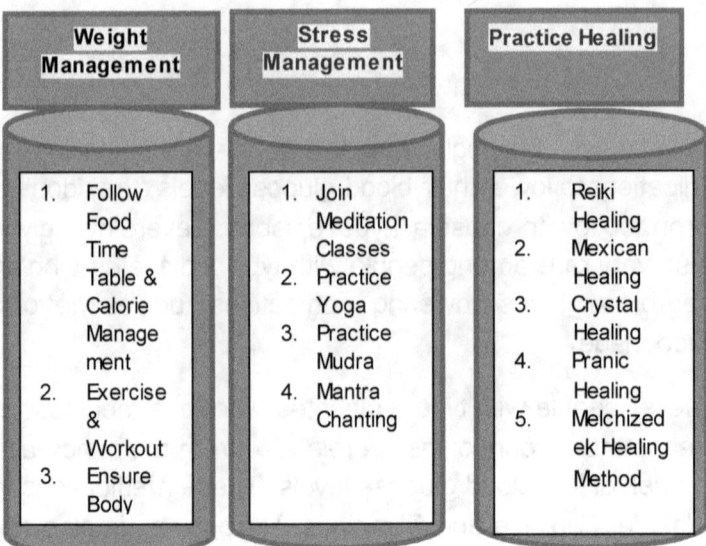

Weight Management	Stress Management	Practice Healing
1. Follow Food Time Table & Calorie Management 2. Exercise & Workout 3. Ensure Body	1. Join Meditation Classes 2. Practice Yoga 3. Practice Mudra 4. Mantra Chanting	1. Reiki Healing 2. Mexican Healing 3. Crystal Healing 4. Pranic Healing 5. Melchizedek Healing Method

Principles of Life

To have a better life and control your diabetics follow below 6 religious principles in life. By following these principles you can cure any diseases not only diabetes.

1. Reiki 5 Principles (By Dr Mikao Usuki – Reiki Founder and Guru)
Just for today, do not be angry

   Just for today, do not worry

   Just for today, be grateful

   Just for today, work hard

   Just for today, be kind to others

   Are you able to solve your issues by worrying or getting angry with others or rude to others? By doing all this you are sending negative energies to your organs. No One has seen tomorrow so what is the purpose of worrying for tomorrow? Live free from worries and stress.

2. Bhagavad Gita (Hindu Religion)
   Do your work/action and do not wait for the results of Karma/actions. You have no right over your actions. Lord Krishna validates your actions and gives you the appropriate results

   Always do your work with full heart. Your customer is god for you. One satisfied customer can multiply your business or generate several customers for your business.

   Also believe no one can change the outcome of your work. Your boss may not give your promotion because of office politics or your teacher may not like you and give less marks in your examination but Lord has seen your results. Believe in god and respect his decision. Outcome of the results will show you a direction and an opportunity for you to improve in your life. Thinks positively and convert your problem as an opportunity for better life.

3. Quran
   You who believe! Seek assistance through patience and prayer surely Allah is with the patient (Quran 2:45 Islam Religion)

   Always cultivate patience in life. Everyone has its own time to show his/her skills. Believe in time. Time is the factor for all your sorrow and disappointments.

4. Buddhism Principles
   Life is filled with vices, things which attempt to bind us to unwholesome ways of living and therefore do the very opposite of cultivate peace, joy, and greater realization in our lives. Among these, the 3 poisons are some of the most powerful. The 3 poisons are:

   i. Greed

ii.　Hatred

iii.　Delusion

These 3 things (Greed, Hatred and Delusion) generate negative energy within our body and mind which may be the cause for any disease within our body. Do not give scope to settle down these negative energies within your body organs.

5.　Jainism Principles
　　The man himself, and he alone, is responsible for all that is good or bad in his life. He cannot absolve himself from the responsibility of experiencing the fruits of his actions.

　　Do not blame anyone in life. Take the responsibility of the problem or challenges you are facing in life. Do not look at the root cause of the problem you are facing. Face it like a university examination. Always give your best shot and do not look into the outcome of it.

6.　Bible (Christianity)
　　Let all bitterness, and wrath, and anger, and clamor, and evil speaking, be put away from you, with all malice: And be ye kind one to another, tenderhearted, forgiving one another, even as God for Christ's sake hath forgiven you." Take a moment and read the story about forgiveness in Matthew 18:23-35 in your Bible.

　　Humans are bound to do mistakes. Forgive them (Friends/Enemies/Hidden Enemies). They made you to learn in life. Make them feel comfortable. If you can't avoid them, nurture them to get good results. Keep your neighbors happy (not only those who lives next door/or work with you also those who are close to you in your mind) and then you can see the illumination in your life.

Appendix A Daily Calorie Needs for Men

Estimates are rounded to the nearest 200 calories. An individual's calorie needs may be higher or lower than these average estimates.

Activity Level/Age	Male/ Sedentary	Male/ Moderately Active	Male/ Active
2	1,000	1,000	1,000
3	1,200	1,400	1,400
4	1,200	1,400	1,600
5	1,200	1,400	1,600
6	1,400	1,600	1,800
7	1,400	1,600	1,800
8	1,400	1,600	2,000
9	1,600	1,800	2,000
10	1,600	1,800	2,200
11	1,800	2,000	2,200
12	1,800	2,200	2,400
13	2,000	2,200	2,600
14	2,000	2,400	2,800
15	2,200	2,600	3,000
16	2,400	2,800	3,200
17	2,400	2,800	3,200
18	2,400	2,800	3,200

19-20	2,600	2,800	3,000
2125-	2400,	2800,	3000,
26-30	2,400	2,600	3,000
31-35	2,400	2,600	3,000
36-40	2,400	2,600	2,800
41-45	2,200	2,600	2,800
46-50	2,200	2,400	2,800
51-55	2,200	2,400	2,800
56-60	2,200	2,400	2,600
61-65	2,000	2,400	2,600
66-70	2,000	2,200	2,600
71-75	2,000	2,200	2,600
76+	2,000	2,200	2,400

Appendix B Daily Calorie Needs for Women

Estimates are rounded to the nearest 200 calories. An individual's calorie needs may be higher or lower than these average estimates.

Activity Level/Age	Female/ Sedentary	Female/ Moderately Active	Female/ Active
2	1,000	1,000	1,000
3	1,000	1,200	1,400
4	1,200	1,400	1,400
5	1,200	1,400	1,600
6	1,200	1,400	1,600
7	1,200	1,600	1,800
8	1,400	1,600	1,800
9	1,400	1,600	1,800
10	1,400	1,800	2,000
11	1,600	1,800	2,000
12	1,600	2,000	2,200
13	1,600	2,000	2,200
14	1,800	2,000	2,400
15	1,800	2,000	2,400
16	1,800	2,000	2,400
17	1,800	2,000	2,400
18	1,800	2,000	2,400
19-20	2,000	2,200	2,400

2125-	2000,	2200,	2400,
26-30	1,800	2,000	2,400
31-35	1,800	2,000	2,200
36-40	1,800	2,000	2,200
41-45	1,800	2,000	2,200
46-50	1,800	2,000	2,200
51-55	1,600	1,800	2,200
56-60	1,600	1,800	2,200
61-65	1,600	1,800	2,000
66-70	1,600	1,800	2,000
71-75	1,600	1,800	2,000
76+	1,600	1,800	2,000

Appendix C List of Yoga for Diabetes

Name of the Yoga	Steps to Practice Yoga
Vrikshasana 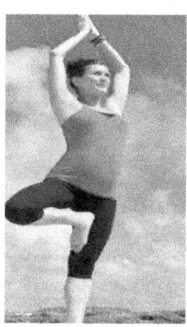	1. Stand straight and keep your feet close to each other. Your knees, legs and hand should be held straight. 2. Now bring your right foot and keep it on your left thigh. Try to make a right angle. If you are unable to keep your foot on the thigh, try to keep your foot on the left leg wherever you feel comfortable and maintain balance. But remember your right toe should point down wards. Your body balance should depend on the left leg. 3. Join your palms and bring them to the middle of your chest and keep the figure pointing upwards. Slowly move your hands overhead. Raise your arms over your head. Your arms should be slightly bent. 4. Stand straight, look in front and try to be relaxed.

5. Stay in this position for about 10 seconds. Breathe normally.
6. Slowly bring your hands in the middle portion of the chest same as before, bring your right leg to the ground and come back in the starting position. - Repeat the same procedure with the other leg.
7. Try to repeat the whole procedure two to three times

Dhanurasana (Bow pose)

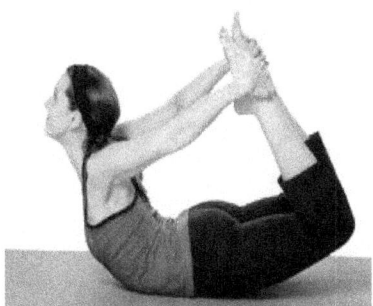

1. Lie on your stomach with your feet hip width apart and your arms by the side of your body.
2. Fold your knees and hold your ankles.
3. Breathing in, lift your chest off the ground and pull your legs up and back.
4. Look straight ahead with a smile on your face. Curve your lips to match the curve of your body.
5. Keep the pose stable while paying attention to your breath. Your body is now taut as a bow.
6. Continue to take long deep breaths as you relax in this pose. But don't get carried away. Do not overdo the stretch.
7. After 15 -20 seconds, as you

exhale, gently bring your legs and chest back to the ground.

8. Release the ankles and relax.

Halasana (Plough Pose)

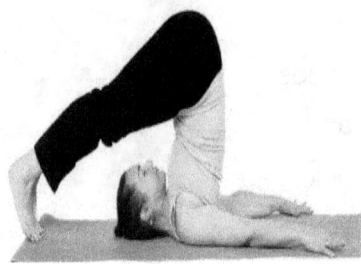

1. Lie on your back with your arms beside you, palms downwards.

As you inhale, use your abdominal muscles to lift your feet off the floor, raising your legs vertically at a 90-degree angle. Continue to breathe normally and supporting your hips and back with your hands, lift them off the ground.

2. Allow your legs to sweep in a 180-degree angle over your head till your toes touch the floor.

3. Your back should be perpendicular to the floor. This may be difficult initially, but make an attempt for a few seconds.

4. Hold this pose and let your body relax more and more with each steady breath.5 after about a minute (a few seconds for

beginners) of resting in this pose, you may gently bring your legs down on exhalation. -Avoid jerking your body, while bringing the legs down

Ardha Matsyendrasana (Half Twist Pose)

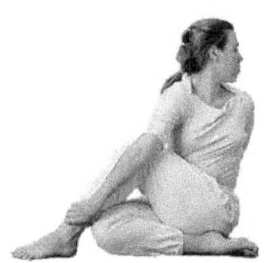

1. Sit on the carpet, stretch the legs straight.
2. Fold the right leg. Keeps the right leg's heel touching the left leg's knee.
3. Take the right hand to back of the waist twisting your trunk, spread palms inside and place it on the carpet.
4. Bring the left hand close to right knee and hold the right leg's ankle or big toe with the left hand.
5. Twist the head and shoulder to right side and look straight to the right shoulder's side (i.e back side).

Appendix D List of Mudra for Diabetes

Surya Mudra [Sun Mudra]:

Steps

Sit or Stand Straight

> Stretch your hands to your front.
> Bend your ring finger of both hands so that it touches the mound of respective thumbs
> Keep the other fingers spread out, apart from each other

Pran Mudra:

Steps

> Sit down in a relaxing position, preferably, Padmasana [Lotus pose], with your eyes closed
> Keep your hands on your sides.
> Bend your little finger and ring finger to touch the thumb.
> Keep the index finger and middle finger straight
> Make sure that you perform this mudra with both the hands.

Apan Mudra [Mudra of Digestion]:

Steps

Sit in Padmasana or Vajrasana.

Keep your hands stretched to your front

Bend your thumb, middle finger, and ring finger in such a way that their tips come together

Keep the little finger and index finger straight

Bend your thumb, middle finger, and ring finger in such a way that their tips come together.

Make sure that you perform this mudra with both the hands.

Gyan Mudra [Mudra of Knowledge]:

Steps:

Choose a sitting position, such as Padmasana, Vajrasana or Sukhasana, depending on your ease of doing so. Those who find it difficult to follow any of the Yoga can opt for sitting relaxingly on a chair.

Keep your eyes closed.

Keep your back straight; head and chest should be held high. Concentrate on your breathing.

Keep your palms on your knees. Palms should face upwards

Bend the index finger to touch the thumb's tip, while the rest of the fingers are kept straight.

Linga Mudra:

Steps:

Sit down in Padmasana, Vajrasana or Sukhasana or choose to stand in Tadasana.

Clasp your hands stretched in front of the body while keeping the fingers intertwined.

The thumb of your left hand should point upward. Circle it with the right thumb and right index finger.

Inhale and exhale normally and maintain the position for 15 minutes

Appendix E Fruits which are Low in Glycemic Load

Fruit	Glycemic Load
Lime	1
Straw berry	1
Apricot	3
Grapefruit	3
Lemon	3
Canteloupe	4
Guava	4
Nectarines	4
Oranges	4
Pear	4
Watermelon	4
Blueberries	5
Peach	5
Plum	5
Apple	6
Pineapple	6
Kiw i	7

Fruit	Glycemic Load
Mango	8
Cherries	9
Prunes	10
Banana	11
Grapes	11
Figs	16
Dates	18
Raisins	28

Appendix F South Indian Food Calorie Table

South Indian Food

Food Item	QTY	Calories (KCAL)
Katori Sambar	1 bowl	121
Cocunut Chutney	1 TBSP	44
Vegetable Uttapham	1	250
Upma	1 bowl	247
Rasam	1 bowl	118
Plain Idli	1	51
Medu Vada	1	103
Masala Dosa	1	415
Plain Dosa	1	120
Neer Dosa	1	105
Chettinad Chicken Curry	1 bowl	497
Avial	1 bowl	130
Puuliyogare	1 plate	261
Chapathi	3 PCS	80
Curd Rice	300 gm	433
Rice Payassam	1 bowl	277

Bisibele bath	300 gms	535
Plain RICE	150 gms	300
Brinjal Sambar	150 gms	199
Banana Porriyal	100 gms	353
Jamoon	40 gms	143
Dry Sweets	1 Piece	80

Appendix G North Indian Food Calorie Table

Starters	Calories (Kcal)
Cucumber raita, 1tbsp	20
Tomato sambal, 1tbsp	20
Mango chutney, 1tbsp	60
Poppadom, each	65
Lime pickle, 1tbsp	70
Onion bhaji, each	190
Vegetable samosa, each	260
Meat samosa, each	320

Main courses	
Tandoori chicken	300
Aloo gobi	330
Vegetable curry	350
Keema madras	450
Aloo saag	500
Beef madras	540
Vegetable biriyani	550
Lamb bhuna	680
Chicken tikka masala	680
Chicken curry	700
Rogan josh	700
Chicken dhansk	720

Appendix H American and Mexican Food Calorie Table

American and Mexican Food

Food	Calories
Starters	
Barbecue ribs	360
Tortilla chips and salsa	515
Chicken wings with barbecue dip	520
Potato skins with sour cream	565
Tortilla chips and guacamole	590
Quesadilla	650
Nachos	1,000
Main courses	
Caesar salad	535
Chicken burrito	600
Chicken enchilada	615
Chicken chimichanga	675
Beef burritos	695

Appendix I British Food Calorie Table

Food	Calories per typical serving
Starters	
Melon	60
Tomato soup	150
Prawn cocktail	350
Breaded mushrooms with dip	370
Pâté and toast	400
Main courses	
Venison in red wine	280
Pork and apple casserole	360
Lancashire hotpot	400
Shepherd's pie	400
Fish pie	450
Beef casserole	490
225g/8oz well-done rump steak with chips	525
Roast beef with trimmings	540
225g/8oz well-done fillet steak and chips	550
Beef Wellington	560
Sausage and mash	585
Toad in the hole	640

Gammon steak and chips	680
Beef stew with dumplings	770
Scampi and chips	820
Steak and kidney pie with chips	820

Desserts

Trifle	270
Lemon meringue pie	305
Spotted dick and custard	435
Apple pie and custard	435
Fruit crumble and custard	475

Appendix J Italian Food Calorie Table

Italian Food	Calories
Starters	
Melon	40
Melon with Parma ham	150
Mozzarella and tomato salad (no ssing)	190
Mixed fish salad	220
Bruschetta	220
Minestrone soup	240
Tuna and bean salad	300
Garlic bread, 4 pieces	400
Main courses	
Spaghetti arrabiata	400
Mushroom risotto	475
Scampi Provençale	500
Cannelloni	500
Ravioli	510
Chicken risotto	550
Spaghetti napoletana	630
Lasagne	650
Spaghetti marinara	690
Spaghetti Bolognese	720
Pizza	750

Spaghetti carbonara	1,020

Desserts

Gelati	140
Cassata	150
Zabaglione	185

Appendix K Chinese Food Calorie Table

Starters

Sesame prawn toasts, per piece	70
Hot and sour soup	80
Prawn wonton, each	80
Spare rib, each	140
Crab and sweetcorn soup	155
Chicken noodle soup	160
Chicken and sweetcorn soup	170
Crispy seaweed	200
Pancake roll	240

Main courses

Chicken in lemon sauce	300
Chicken and pineapple	310
Beef in oyster sauce	340
Beef in yellow bean sauce	360
Beef with green peppers and black bean sauce	380
Chicken and cashew nuts	380
Chicken chop suey	425
Sweet and sour chicken	480
Crispy duck, four pancakes	800
Prawns balls (10) in batter with sweet and sour sauce	1,200

Appendix L Singaporean Food Calorie Table

Murtabak (Mutton)	1102 kcal
Nasi Goreng Sayur	920 kcal
Nasi Briyani Chicken	877 kcal
Pad Thai	840 kcal
Lontong with Sayur Lodeh	798 kcal
Char Kway Teow	730 kcal
Deep Fried Fish Beehoon Soup (with evaporated milk)	700 kcal
Laksa	697 kcal
Beef Horfun	695 kcal
Curry Noodles	694 kcal
Mee Siam	692 kcal
Mee Goreng	677 kcal
Seafood Claypot Noodles	656 kcal
Beef Ball Kway Teow Soup	650 kcal
Kway Chap	617 kcal
Chicken Rice	605 kcal
Char Siew Rice	604 kcal
Duck Rice Braised	585 kcal
Lor Mee	595 kcal
Fried Carrot Cake (with Dark Sauce)	580 kcal
Chye Peng (1 stir fried meat + 2 veg + rice)	(2 pieces) 576 kcal
Roti Prata with Egg	576 kcal

Appendix M Indonesian Food Calorie Table

Indonesian Food	Servings	Calories (Kcal)
Kue Lupis	1 Cake	100
Nasi Uduk	1/2 cup	116
Cap Cay	1 plate	130
Lamb Curry	1 cup	257
Perkedel	50 g	123
Sambal Goreng Ati Kentang	1 cup	127
Krecek Sayur	3 cup	249
Pastel	1 piece	123
Bakpia	1 piece	68
Terong	1 cup	25
Kroket	1 piece	146
Ikan Mas	1 piece	172
Ketan	1 piece	240
Pempek	200 gms	384
Leupet Ketan	1 piece	240
Tape Ketan Hitam	1 cup	166
Tape Ketan Putih	1 cup	172
Kue Apem	1 piece	187
Telur Asin (Bebek)	100 g	195
Lemper	1 piece	95

Appendix N Malaysian Food Calorie Table

Food	Kcal
Nasi Lemak	644
Fied Chicken	290
The Tarik	81
Roti Cannai	359
Roti Telur	414
2 Pcs Curry Puff	256
Chapathi Green Gravy	166
2 Half Boil Egg/Plain Bread	227
Plain Sardine Sandwiches	71
Mamak Mee Goreng	660
Prawn Mee Soup	293
Lor Mee	383
Mee Rebus	556
Mee Hailam	277
Wantan Mee Soup	217
Fried Meehoon/Noodle	510
Wantan Mee Dry	409
Penang Laksa	436
Noodle Soup	381
1 pc Cucur Udang	144
1 pc Yau Car Kuih	292
1 pc Goreng Pisang	129

Appendix O Alcoholic Beverage Calorie Table

Beverage

Description	Quantity	KCAL
Red Wine	1 Glass (5 oz)	105
White Wine Dry	1 Glass (5 oz)	97
White Wine Sweet	1 Glass (5 oz)	135
Champagne	1 Glass (5 oz)	70
Screw Driver	1 Glass (5 oz)	180
Margarita	1 Glass (5 oz)	157
Whisky	1 Glass (5 oz)	125
Bacardi	1 Glass (5 oz)	110
Vodka (Neat)	1 Shot	65
Rum (Neat)	1 Shot	66
Tequila (Neat)	1 Shot	65
Brandy (Neat)	1 Shot	64
Scotch (Neat)	1 Shot	64
Beer Lighr	330 ml	100
Beer Regular	330 ml	146
Gin (Neat)	1 Shot	65

Appendix P Milk Product Calorie Table

Milk Product	Quantity	KCAL
Milk	1 Glass	100
Condensed Milk	1 Glass	320
Skimmed Milk	1 Glass	45
Skimmed Butter Milk	1 Glass	60
Curds/Yoghurt	1 Cup	60
Khoa	1/2 Cup	205
Butter	1 Tbsp	120
Ice Cream	1 Scoop	114
Shredded Cheese	1/2 Cup	150
Blue Cheese	1/2 Cup	100
Cheese	1/2 Cup	82
Cottage Cheese	1tbsp	16
Ghee	2tbsp(10 gm)	120

www.ingramcontent.com/pod-product-compliance
Lightning Source LLC
Chambersburg PA
CBHW062343280526
45787CB00012B/713

* 9 7 8 1 5 2 2 8 7 0 3 9 5 *